Breaking

Free

Breaking Free:

Unshackling Yourself from Masturbation for Holistic Well-being and Personal Transformation.

Bruce P. FRYE

Copyright

Dedication

To my mindful loved ones, who have everlastingly been my inspiration and my sincerely strong organization. Much obliged to you for engaging me to seek after my dreams and for ceaselessly staying nearby, during the most inconvenient times. This book is committed to you, with all my fondness and appreciation.

Contents

CHAPTER ONE

Introduction

The phenomenon of excessive masturbation, often marginalized or downplayed, reveals itself as a subtle yet pervasive force with profound effects on an individual's well-being.

Far beyond being merely an exercise in perceived indulgence, excessive masturbation intricately weaves itself into the fabric of both physical and mental health, demanding recognition and understanding to be at the forefront of any comprehensive wellness journey.

At its core, excessive masturbation goes beyond isolated events, seeping into various aspects of a person's life.

This acknowledgment forms a symbiotic relationship with the intricate webs of physical and mental health that collectively shape an individual's condition.

To embark on a transformative journey toward complete wellness, individuals are called to delve deeper into their behaviors, recognizing their impact on overall well-being.

The intersection of excessive metabolism and physical health unveils itself through a cascade of effects, including a decrease in vital neurotransmitters, disruption of hormonal balance, and depletion of essential energy.

The dynamic dance of dopamine and serotonin, crucial neurotransmitters, becomes a neurological fragility susceptible to decay when disturbed by excessive release during hypersexual episodes. Establishing a hormonal balance, especially during orgasmic peaks, proves essential for overall well-being. This complex interaction extends beyond immediate physiological reactions, influencing broader physiological responses and dynamics within the body.

Simultaneously, excessive masturbation poses a potential threat to mental health by contributing to elevated stress levels, disturbances in sleep patterns, and an increased risk of addiction. This cycle, if left unchecked, can lead to substantial damage to one's mental well-being.

Recognizing and understanding these complexities goes beyond a mere qualitative exercise; it marks the initiation of a profound journey toward complete wellness. This journey involves peeling back the layers of one's physical and mental environment, comprehending the intricate factors at play, and acknowledging their collective impact on overall health.

This knowledge serves as an illuminating guide, paving the way for a well-balanced existence where individuals can make informed decisions, adopt healthy habits, and foster a lifestyle that nurtures both body and mind.

In essence, it is an exploration that transcends the surface, offering a holistic perspective on the intricate interplay between excessive masturbation and well-being.

Understanding the consequences of excessive masturbation.

1. **Fatigue and Energy Drain**

Understanding the consequences of excessive masturbation involves scrutinizing its acute effects on physical and psychological well-being. Focusing on "fatigue and energy expenditure," we explore how excessive sex leads to physical exhaustion, depletes vital energy, and affects overall energy levels.

This brief insight into sex, a significant influencer of both energy and well-being, spans various dimensions.

Excessive masturbation, marked by an unrelenting preoccupation with sexual thoughts and behaviors, takes a toll on the physical body. Frequent and intense sexual activity goes beyond momentary fatigue, impacting daily life and hindering routine activities.

Depleting vital energy is a significant outcome. While orgasm initially boosts energy through neurotransmitters and hormones, excess release taxes the body's energy reserves, contributing to weariness. Mental processes are not spared, as excessive masturbation's fixation induces mental fatigue, leading to concentration challenges and disrupted sleep patterns.

The cyclical nature of excessive masturbation, with intense bouts followed by recovery, induces fluctuations in energy levels, adding instability to overall well-being.

Recognizing these complexities is vital, urging individuals to make informed decisions, manage fatigue, and embrace a holistic approach to well-being considering the intricate relationship between excessive masturbation and energy expenditure.

a. Physiological Impact:

Masturbation acts as a trigger for neurotransmitters, particularly dopamine and serotonin, crucial for shaping feelings of pleasure and satisfaction in the brain. These neurotransmitters are integral for overall well-being, contributing to the maintenance of a positive state of mind. However, the crux of the matter lies in the delicate balance of these neurotransmitters.

Under normal and healthy conditions, the release of dopamine and serotonin fosters feelings of happiness and satisfaction, playing pivotal roles in mood regulation, motivation, and overall emotional well-being. Nevertheless, repeated and has the potential to disrupt this delicate equilibrium.

Picture these neurotransmitters as a limited resource, akin to a well-preserved reservoir. With each instance of masturbation, the demand for dopamine and serotonin surges. If this reservoir is frequently depleted, it appears that the consequence could be a degradation of these essential neuronal reserves.

This degradation carries implications for sustained energy levels. Envision the brain as an electrical plant reliant on a steady supply of these neurotransmitters to function optimally.

If these substances are consistently absorbed without adequate recovery time, the delicate balance may shift, resulting in feelings of fatigue and diminished energy levels throughout the body.

An apt analogy would be that of a depleting battery. Dopamine and serotonin act as potent molecules governing cognitive and emotional processes. The parallel with lies in the inability of the battery to recharge adequately, making it prone to rapid discharge and subsequently impacting the overall energy output of the system.

Understanding this intricate balance provides valuable insights into how can influence an individual's energy levels. It underscores the significance of moderation for sustained well-being, emphasizing the need to be mindful of the potential consequences of disrupting the delicate interplay of neurotransmitters in the pursuit of pleasure and satisfaction.

b. Hormonal Fluctuations:

The intricate dance of sexual arousal and orgasm orchestrates the release of hormones such as prolactin and oxytocin, contributing to both the physiological and emotional aspects of the experience.

Prolactin, often referred to as the "satisfaction hormone," fosters a profound sense of fulfillment, while oxytocin, known as the "love hormone," facilitates emotional bonding.

However, this delicate hormonal dance can face disruption through frequent masturbation. Envision these hormones as skilled dancers performing in perfect harmony.

With each instance of masturbation, there is an increased demand for the release of prolactin and oxytocin.

Now, picture these dancers being called to perform repeatedly without sufficient intermissions. The continuous overstimulation of these hormonal responses, especially through frequent masturbation, disrupts the delicate equilibrium that governs their release.

This disruption can lead to an imbalance in hormonal levels, potentially resulting in pervasive fatigue.

In essence, the hormonal system, akin to a finely tuned orchestra, necessitates periods of rest and recovery to maintain its delicate balance. Frequent masturbation without adequate intervals for hormonal equilibrium may contribute to a sense of pervasive fatigue, impacting both physical and emotional well-being.

This analogy vividly illustrates how the intricate hormonal dance, when disrupted through overstimulation, plays a significant role in influencing the overall energy levels and vitality of an individual.

c. Energy Expenditure:

The physical act of masturbation, coupled with its associated physiological responses, places a notable demand on the body's energy resources.

It's comparable to engaging in a physical exercise that requires stamina and effort.

Similar to an athlete needing recovery time after an intense workout, the body also requires a period of recuperation after the energy expenditure involved in masturbation.

Imagine the body as an energy bank, with each instance of masturbation akin to a withdrawal. Without allowing sufficient time for recovery, frequent engagement in this activity can lead to a cumulative depletion of energy resources.

This analogy highlights how, much like any physical exertion, masturbation requires energy, and a lack of adequate recovery intervals may contribute to an overall sense of energy depletion.

Understanding this dynamic emphasizes the importance of moderation and recognizing the need for the body to restore its energy reserves. It underscores the significance of balancing sexual activities with the body's natural ability to recover, promoting overall well-being and sustained vitality.

This awareness encourages individuals to approach sexual practices with a mindful consideration of their energy dynamics, fostering a healthy equilibrium for long-term physical and mental wellness.

2. Impact on the Nervous System

Masturbation acts as a trigger for the sympathetic nervous system, the segment of our autonomic nervous system responsible for the "fight or flight" response.

This physiological reaction prepares the body to confront or escape from perceived threats. While crucial in emergencies, frequent activation through masturbation can lead to overstimulation.

Visualize the sympathetic nervous system as a vigilant guardian, always poised for action. When activated by masturbation, it readies the body for perceived challenges or excitement.

However, when this response is triggered repeatedly without sufficient intervals, it results in a persistent state of overstimulation. This continuous heightened alertness, resembling the body being kept in a perpetual state of readiness, significantly contributes to feelings of exhaustion.

Picture it as a car engine constantly revving at high RPMs. While sustainable for short bursts, this level of activation becomes unsustainable and fatiguing when prolonged.

Similarly, the persistent stimulation of the sympathetic nervous system without adequate recovery time may lead to a state of overstimulation, intensifying alertness and ultimately contributing to a sense of physical and mental exhaustion.

Understanding this physiological response sheds light on the potential consequences of frequent masturbation on overall well-being.

It emphasizes the importance of allowing the body to return to a state of balance and relaxation, promoting a healthier equilibrium for sustained energy levels.

This insight underscores the need for individuals to be mindful of the impact of their sexual practices on the body's physiological responses and to incorporate adequate recovery time for optimal well-being.

3. Cortisol Levels:

The stress hormone cortisol, a pivotal player in the body's response to heightened arousal or stress, is released during moments of intense stimulation, including those experienced during masturbation.

In a typical scenario, cortisol helps regulate various physiological processes, preparing the body to cope with stressors.

However, can lead to a persistent elevation of cortisol levels. Envision cortisol as a signal that prompts the body to gear up for challenges.

When this signal is activated frequently without adequate recovery time, it subjects the body to prolonged stress.

The continuous elevation of cortisol levels contributes to an extended state of heightened stress, fostering subsequent fatigue.

Picture it as keeping the body in a chronic state of alertness, akin to being in a constant state of high alert.

Just as prolonged stress in daily life can lead to fatigue, the persistent elevation of cortisol due to may contribute to a sense of prolonged stress, ultimately impacting overall energy levels and well-being.

Understanding this hormonal aspect sheds light on how can influence the body's stress response, emphasizing the importance of moderation and allowing the body sufficient time for recovery to maintain a healthy hormonal balance.

This insight underscores the need for individuals to be mindful of the potential impact of frequent masturbation on cortisol levels and the subsequent implications for overall well-being.

4. Sleep Disruptions

Frequent masturbation, especially when done in close proximity to bedtime, can significantly impact sleep patterns. Consider the period leading up to sleep as a crucial phase for the body to transition into a state of rest and recovery.

Engaging in masturbation close to bedtime may stimulate the nervous system and release hormones that ideally should be in a state of decline to promote restful sleep. The resulting heightened arousal and activation of physiological responses can disrupt the natural progression into a restful sleep state.

Visualize trying to wind down for the night, but your body is still in an alert and active mode. This disruption in the natural sleep cycle can lead to inadequate or disturbed sleep, reducing the overall quality of rest.

The consequences of this sleep disturbance extend beyond the night, intricately connecting with daily activities and vitality.

Picture a disrupted sleep pattern as a ripple effect that permeates the following day. Inadequate sleep is associated with decreased overall energy levels, impacting an individual's ability to fully engage in daily activities.

The interconnectedness of sleep and vitality underscores the importance of considering the timing and frequency of masturbation in relation to sleep, emphasizing the need for a balanced approach to maintain overall well-being.

This awareness highlights the role of mindful choices in optimizing sleep quality and, consequently, supporting sustained vitality.

5. Chronic Fatigue Syndrome

There are reports suggesting a correlation between chronic and the manifestation of symptoms resembling Chronic Fatigue Syndrome (CFS).

Chronic Fatigue Syndrome is characterized by persistent, unexplained fatigue that is not alleviated by rest and is often accompanied by other symptoms like impaired concentration and muscle pain.

The intricate relationship between the physiological and psychological strain induced by frequent sexual activity suggests a potential contribution to the development of symptoms akin to CFS.

Envision the body as a finely tuned instrument, and as a continuous strain on its intricate mechanisms.

Frequent engagement in sexual activity, without adequate intervals for recovery, may subject the body to a persistent state of physiological and psychological stress.

This chronic stress, both physical and mental, can lead to a cascade of effects on the body's overall well-being. The potential manifestation of symptoms resembling CFS highlights the importance of recognizing the intricate balance required for sustained health and the potential consequences of excessive activities on the body's resilience.

Understanding this correlation emphasizes the need for moderation and self-awareness in sexual practices, considering the holistic impact on both physical and mental health.

It encourages individuals to be attuned to their bodies, recognizing signs of potential strain, and adopting practices that promote overall well-being and vitality.

This awareness underscores the importance of a balanced approach to sexual activities, allowing for adequate recovery and fostering a state of equilibrium for optimal health.

6. Impact on Daily Activities and Overall Vitality

The consequences of frequent and extend beyond the immediate physical act, significantly impacting an individual's motivation, productivity, and overall well-being.

Reduced Motivation and Productivity

The fatigue induced by creates a significant hurdle in maintaining motivation and productivity in daily tasks. Imagine trying to navigate through work, hobbies, or social activities with a depleted energy reserve.

The challenge becomes apparent as the body struggles to summon the necessary drive, making engagement in these activities a more difficult endeavor.

Physical and Mental Sluggishness

The confluence of physical exhaustion and potential disruptions to mental well-being culminates in an overarching sensation of sluggishness.

This lethargy is not confined to the immediate post-masturbation period but lingers throughout the day.

Picture trying to operate with both body and mind in a state of reduced alertness and responsiveness. The result is a pervasive feeling of sluggishness that affects an individual's sustained energy levels, hindering optimal functioning.

Understanding these intricate details provides individuals with a holistic perspective on the far-reaching impact of excessive masturbation.

Armed with this knowledge, individuals can make informed decisions about their sexual practices and implement strategies that prioritize balanced physical and mental well-being.

This awareness serves as a guiding force, empowering individuals to adopt practices that

promote vitality and sustained energy throughout
their   daily   lives

CHAPTER TWO

Recognizing the Signs

Identifying Indicators of Excessive Masturbation.

In the quest for a wholesome connection with one's sexuality, it becomes paramount to immerse oneself in the nuanced landscape of signs that may indicate excessive masturbation.

This exploration transcends the mere physical act, delving into the intricate realms of emotions and behaviors. It seeks to provide a comprehensive understanding of an individual's overall well-being, weaving together the intricate threads of physical and mental experiences.

Physical Aspects:

Discerning signs on a physical level entails attentiveness to the body's responses and cues. These may encompass shifts in energy levels, disturbances in sleep patterns, and potential indications of fatigue.

A heightened sensitivity to how the body physically reacts to sexual activities offers valuable insights into whether these practices align with the body's innate rhythms and natural balance.

Emotional Indicators

Emotional well-being intricately intertwines with sexual health. Indicators of may manifest as fluctuations in mood, heightened anxiety, or disproportionate stress responses.

Scrutinizing these emotional nuances empowers individuals to assess the influence of their sexual practices on their mental and emotional states. This observation serves as a crucial compass in navigating the delicate interplay between emotional well-being and sexual health.

Behavioral Changes:

Behaviors often serve as visible markers of underlying issues. Compulsive behaviors, a diminished ability to control the frequency or intensity of masturbation, or neglecting daily responsibilities due to preoccupation with sexual activities are significant behavioral indicators.

Recognizing these changes provides individuals with a mirror to assess whether their sexual practices align with a healthy and balanced lifestyle.

This multifaceted exploration of signs extends beyond a mere checklist, offering a holistic approach to understanding one's sexual health. It encourages individuals to be attuned to the interconnected nature of physical, emotional, and behavioral aspects, fostering a more nuanced and comprehensive perspective on the intricate relationship between sexuality and overall well-being.

This depth of understanding serves as a valuable compass in navigating the landscape of sexual health and its profound impact on one's holistic well-being.

Physical Signs:

Fatigue and Physical Exhaustion:

can induce a persistent sense of tiredness and physical exhaustion, significantly impacting the body's overall energy levels

Depletion of Neurotransmitters:

Masturbation triggers the release of neurotransmitters, such as dopamine and serotonin, contributing to feelings of pleasure and satisfaction. However, frequent and excessive release of these neurotransmitters can lead to their depletion.

This depletion may result in a sense of fatigue as the body grapples with maintaining the delicate balance necessary for sustained energy. The intricate dance of neurotransmitters highlights the importance of moderation, ensuring a harmonious interplay for optimal well-being.

Hormonal Fluctuations:

Sexual arousal and orgasm entail the release of hormones like prolactin and oxytocin. Overstimulation of these hormonal responses, particularly with frequent masturbation, has the potential to disrupt the delicate hormonal equilibrium.

This disruption may contribute to a persistent feeling of tiredness and physical exhaustion.

The intricate hormonal interplay underscores the importance of moderation in sexual activities, allowing for the maintenance of a balanced hormonal environment for overall well-being.

Energy Expenditure:

Engaging in masturbation and the associated physiological responses demand a considerable amount of energy. Frequent involvement in this activity without adequate recovery time can lead to an overall depletion of energy resources. This depletion manifests as fatigue, affecting the body's ability to sustain optimal energy levels. The continuous strain on energy resources highlights the importance of recognizing the need for moderation and sufficient recovery intervals to maintain overall vitality.

Impact on the Nervous System:

Masturbation stimulates the sympathetic nervous system, triggering the "fight or flight" response. Frequent activation of this response can lead to overstimulation, causing the body to remain in a heightened state of alertness.

This overstimulation contributes significantly to physical exhaustion and a pervasive sense of tiredness.

The persistent activation of the sympathetic nervous system emphasizes the importance of allowing the body to return to a state of balance and relaxation, promoting a healthier equilibrium for sustained energy levels.

Cortisol Levels:

The stress hormone cortisol is released during moments of heightened arousal. may elevate cortisol levels, leading to prolonged stress on the body and subsequent physical fatigue.

The persistent elevation of cortisol levels underscores the need for moderation in sexual practices, allowing for the body to recover and maintain a healthy hormonal balance for overall well-being

Sleep Disruptions

Frequent masturbation, especially close to bedtime, can disrupt sleep patterns. Inadequate or disturbed sleep can result in decreased overall energy levels, contributing to feelings of fatigue during waking hours.

The intricate relationship between sexual activities and sleep underscores the importance of considering timing and frequency to promote a balanced approach that supports optimal energy levels and overall well-being.

Chronic Fatigue Syndrome Correlation

Some individuals engaging in chronic and have reported symptoms resembling chronic fatigue syndrome (CFS).

While the exact link is complex, it suggests that the physiological and psychological strain from frequent sexual activity may contribute to CFS-like symptoms, further intensifying feelings of fatigue.

Understanding the nuanced interplay of neurotransmitters, hormones, energy expenditure, nervous system activation, and potential correlations with chronic fatigue syndrome provides insight into how can lead to a persistent sense of fatigue and physical exhaustion.

This recognition serves as a crucial step in addressing and mitigating these effects for overall well-being.

It emphasizes the importance of a balanced approach to sexual activities, considering the potential impact on both physical and mental health, and underscores the need for self-awareness in promoting sustained vitality.

Emotional and Behavioral Signs:

Increased Anxiety or Stress:

Escalating levels of anxiety or stress that appear disproportionate to daily challenges can serve as a significant indicator of an imbalance in one's relationship with masturbation.

This heightened emotional response may suggest that the act of masturbation is contributing to, rather than alleviating, emotional well-being.

Recognizing such emotional signals becomes essential in fostering a mindful and balanced approach to sexual practices, promoting a harmonious integration of physical and emotional health. This awareness allows individuals to make informed choices that prioritize overall well-being and emotional equilibrium.

Compulsive Behavior

A compulsive urge to engage in masturbation, accompanied by a diminished ability to control the frequency or intensity of this behavior, signifies potential issues with self-regulation.

The persistent and uncontrollable nature of this urge may point to a deeper emotional or psychological dependency on the act. Recognizing these signs becomes crucial in addressing the underlying factors contributing to compulsive behavior, fostering a journey towards healthier self-regulation and overall well-being

Neglect of Responsibilities:

Neglecting daily responsibilities, such as work, studies, or social commitments, due to preoccupation with masturbation indicates an unhealthy shift in priorities.

This behavioral sign suggests that the act of masturbation has taken precedence over essential life responsibilities, impacting overall functioning and well-being.

Recognizing this imbalance becomes essential in restoring a healthy perspective on priorities, fostering a more sustainable approach to both sexual practices and daily life commitments.

Emotional Disproportion:

The key lies in recognizing when anxiety or stress becomes disproportionate to the challenges faced in daily life. If masturbation is contributing to heightened emotional distress rather than serving as a healthy outlet, it may indicate a need for reevaluation. This awareness empowers individuals to assess the impact of their sexual practices on emotional well-being and prompts thoughtful consideration of adjustments to foster a more balanced and beneficial relationship with masturbation.

Compulsive Patterns

The term "compulsive" implies a lack of control over one's actions. If the urge to masturbate becomes a repetitive and uncontrollable pattern, it may point towards a reliance on the behavior as a coping mechanism or a means of escape. Recognizing this compulsive pattern is crucial, as it suggests a need for deeper introspection and potentially seeking support to address underlying emotional or psychological factors contributing to the behavior.

Prioritization of Masturbation over Responsibilities

Neglecting essential responsibilities due to preoccupation with masturbation raises concerns about the impact of this behavior on daily functioning. It suggests a potential interference with work, academic pursuits, or social interactions, warranting attention and intervention.

Recognizing these signs prompts individuals to assess the balance between sexual activities and life commitments, encouraging a more holistic and sustainable approach that prioritizes overall well-being.

Addressing these Signs:

Open Communication:

- Initiating open and non-judgmental communication about these signs with oneself or a trusted confidant is a crucial first step.

Acknowledging the presence of these indicators is the foundation for addressing any potential concerns.

This self-awareness and willingness to communicate pave the way for a more informed and supportive approach to navigate the complexities of one's relationship with masturbation and overall well-being.

- Professional Guidance

Seeking the guidance of a mental health professional can provide valuable insights into the underlying emotional or psychological factors contributing to these signs.

Professional support can offer effective strategies for coping and behavior modification. This proactive step towards seeking assistance underscores the importance of addressing the multifaceted aspects of one's relationship with masturbation, promoting mental and emotional well-being.

- Behavioral Modification:

Implementing intentional strategies for behavioral modification, such as setting boundaries and engaging in alternative activities, can assist in breaking compulsive patterns and restoring a healthier balance in one's life. Recognizing and addressing emotional and behavioral signs associated with masturbation is essential for fostering a balanced and fulfilling life.

By understanding these nuances, individuals can embark on a journey of self-discovery and make informed decisions to enhance their overall well-being.

This proactive approach empowers individuals to cultivate a mindful and harmonious relationship with their sexuality, contributing to a more holistic and fulfilling lifestyle.

Interpersonal relationship

1. Strained Relationships

may lead to emotional withdrawal, impacting the quality of interpersonal relationships. The heightened focus on individual sexual activities may divert attention and emotional energy away from meaningful connections with others.

Recognizing this potential impact highlights the importance of maintaining a balanced approach to sexual practices, ensuring that relationships with oneself and others thrive in a supportive and emotionally connected environment.

2. Communication Breakdown

Difficulties in communicating openly about sexual habits may contribute to misunderstandings and a breakdown in intimacy.

A lack of transparent communication regarding sexual preferences, boundaries, or concerns can create barriers to understanding between partners.

Recognizing the importance of open and honest dialogue fosters a healthier sexual environment, promoting trust, intimacy, and mutual understanding within the relationship.

Navigating the Path to Awareness and Balance

Recognizing the signs of is the initial step toward cultivating awareness. Individuals can embark on a journey to balance by fostering an open dialogue about their sexual health, seeking support when needed, and embracing strategies that promote a harmonious integration of sexuality into their overall well-being.

This holistic approach allows for a healthier, more fulfilling relationship with one's own body and sexuality.

It encourages self-reflection, open communication, and proactive steps to achieve a balanced and satisfying connection with one's sexual well-being.

Chapter 3

The Decisive Path to Change

Embarking on the transformative odyssey demands a profound recognition of the imperative for change, signifying a pivotal stride that constructs the groundwork for embracing an unequivocal path towards a novel and refined reality.

This pivotal acknowledgment acts as the instigator for the subsequent metamorphosis, propelling individuals towards a heightened sense of fulfillment and a purposeful existence.

Let us intricately explore the fundamental facets of this transformative process, where the intertwining dynamics of self-awareness and unwavering determination emerge as the vanguards, intricately laying the mosaic for favorable change and fostering personal growth.

Acknowledging the Need for Transformation

Initiating a process of deep self-reflection to gain insight into existing patterns and behaviors that warrant transformation.

Embarking on a journey of self-reflection is a profound and introspective process that involves delving into one's thoughts, emotions, and behaviors to gain a deeper understanding of oneself.

In the context of acknowledging the need for transformation, this step is crucial for recognizing existing patterns and behaviors that may be contributing to the desire for change.

Key Components of Self-Reflection:

1. Identification of Patterns:

- Commencing the transformative journey entails the meticulous identification of recurrent patterns entwined within one's thoughts, emotions, and actions.

When confronting excessive masturbation, the initial step involves a discerning recognition of the instances, motives, and associated emotions or triggers propelling this behavior.

Example: Embark on this introspective venture by keenly observing and acknowledging the repetitive patterns in your thoughts, emotions, and actions linked to excessive masturbation.

Consider maintaining a journal to meticulously document occurrences of this behavior. Delve into details, noting the timings, situations, and emotional states entwined with these occurrences.

This reflective practice serves as a compass for navigating the nuanced landscape of personal transformation.

2. Exploration of Motivations:

Plunging into the motivations steering present behaviors stands as an indispensable facet of the transformative process.

This necessitates posing incisive queries such as, "What propels me to partake in these actions?" or "Do underlying emotions or unmet needs exert influence on my behavior?" Unraveling the root causes unveils insights into the psychological dimensions that warrant attention.

Example: Initiate a profound exploration into the motivations underpinning your existing behaviors. Pose penetrating questions like, "What drives me to engage in excessive masturbation?"

and "Are there underlying emotions or unmet needs influencing my behavior?

This investigative journey may unearth connections between the behavior and deeper psychological facets, fostering a nuanced understanding essential for personal evolution.

3. Examining Coping Mechanisms:

Numerous behaviors, encompassing the realm of excessive masturbation, often emerge as coping mechanisms for navigating stress, anxiety, or other challenges.

Engaging in self-reflection entails delving into alternative and healthier coping mechanisms while comprehending the reasons specific behaviors have evolved into default responses to stressors.

Example: Acknowledge that behaviors, including excessive masturbation, frequently function as coping mechanisms amid stress or anxiety.

Embark on an exploration of alternative, healthier coping mechanisms like mindfulness, exercise, or creative activities.

Grasp the intricacies of why certain behaviors have assumed the role of default responses to stressors, evaluating their efficacy in fostering overall well-being.

This introspective journey acts as a compass for steering towards healthier coping strategies.

4. Assessment of Emotional States:

The pivotal recognition of emotional states intertwined with specific behaviors forms a cornerstone of the transformative journey.

In the context of excessive masturbation, an individual may unveil connections to feelings of loneliness, stress, or boredom. This heightened awareness serves as a catalyst for directly addressing these underlying emotions, surpassing reliance on the behavior as a coping mechanism.

Example: Cultivate a keen observance of the emotional states entangled with excessive masturbation. Should you discern a correlation between this behavior and feelings of loneliness, stress, or boredom, acknowledge these emotional triggers.

This heightened awareness empowers you to confront the underlying emotions head-on, paving the way for the cultivation of healthier coping strategies. This deliberate shift marks a significant stride towards holistic well-being.

Why Engage in Self-Reflection?

Embarking on the odyssey of personal development and transformation, the art of self-reflection surfaces as a potent and indispensable tool.

This chapter endeavors to delve into the profound rationales behind advocating for active participation in self-reflection and elucidates the transformative impact it wields upon the lives of individuals.

1. Self-Understanding:

- Plunging into the depths of self-discovery empowers individuals to discern patterns and motivations that govern their behavior.

This intricate process demands astute observation and introspection, unraveling the complexities woven into one's thoughts, emotions, and actions.

By keeping a reflective journal, an individual may uncover recurring patterns of linked to specific times of the day or emotional states.

This self-awareness forms the foundation for understanding the driving forces behind their behavior.

2. Empowerment for Change:

Grasping the root causes of behavior bequeaths a profound sense of empowerment. Armed with insights garnered through self-reflection, individuals become adept at making informed decisions geared towards positive change.

By recognizing that often functions as a coping mechanism for stress, an individual gain the agency to consciously opt for alternative, healthier coping strategies.

This newfound empowerment serves as the catalyst for breaking free from less desirable habits, ushering in a transformative journey towards holistic well-being.

3. Healthier Coping Strategies:

Embracing self-reflection serves as an invitation to explore alternative coping mechanisms, ushering in the substitution of less healthy habits.

This proactive approach to managing stress and challenges becomes a cornerstone of overall well-being.

Upon recognizing that functions as a default response to boredom, an individual may embark on exploring creative activities or exercise as healthier alternatives.

This intentional shift towards positive coping mechanisms lays the foundation for a more balanced and resilient lifestyle, marking a transformative stride in the pursuit of holistic well-being.

4. Emotional Well-Being:

The intricate process of self-reflection becomes a gateway for individuals to recognize and proactively address emotional triggers.

Through heightened awareness of these triggers, individuals can take intentional steps to bolster overall emotional health and resilience.

Discovering a link between feelings of loneliness and prompts individuals to confront the underlying emotional need for connection.

This heightened awareness becomes a catalyst for fostering healthier relationships and nurturing emotional well-being.

Active participation in self-reflection, coupled with the embrace of these intentional steps, unfurls a journey of personal growth and heightened self-awareness. The prospect of positive transformations in various facets of life not only becomes conceivable but also within reach.

In the forthcoming chapters, a more in-depth exploration of practical strategies and insights will guide individuals on their path to holistic well-being, offering motivational insight to fuel their transformative endeavors.

Motivational Insights: Igniting the Flames of Change

In the relentless pursuit of personal transformation, the beacon of motivational insights stands as the propelling force that thrusts individuals forward on the arduous yet rewarding path of change.

This section intricately delves into key perspectives that illuminate the profound reasons why embarking on this transformative journey holds unparalleled significance.

1. Enhanced Well-being:

The profound realization that transformative change is inherently intertwined with an elevated state of overall well-being serves as the bedrock of motivation.

This encompasses not only enhancements in physical health but also the cultivation of heightened mental clarity and a profound sense of vitality.

Wholeheartedly embracing change through the adoption of healthier habits, including the management of excessive masturbation, becomes a contributory force towards reduced fatigue, elevated energy levels, and an overarching sense of well-being.

This synergistic approach sets the stage for a transformative journey that extends beyond the physical realm, encompassing the holistic spectrum of one's well-being.

2. Positive Relationships:

- The profound recognition of the positive ripple effect on personal relationships emerges as a potent motivator. Acknowledging that individual growth contributes to more meaningful and fulfilling connections with others underscores the paramount importance of personal transformation.

Liberating oneself from detrimental habits holds the potential to usher in improved communication, heightened emotional availability, and a deeper connection with loved ones.

This transformative shift fosters stronger and more positive relationships, exemplifying the profound impact that personal growth can have on the tapestry of human connections.

3. Increased Productivity:

The acknowledgment of the potential for breaking free from detrimental habits to amplify productivity and effectiveness in daily tasks and endeavors stands as a formidable motivator.

The enticing prospect of reclaiming time and energy for more meaningful pursuits becomes a compelling driving force.

Surpassing habits such as holds the key to liberating precious time and mental energy.

This newfound freedom allows individuals to channel their focus and efforts into activities that substantially contribute to both personal and professional growth, ushering in a transformative wave of purposeful living.

4. Emotional Resilience:

Embracing change as a pathway to constructing emotional resilience equips individuals with the essential tools to navigate life's myriad challenges with a more balanced and composed mindset.

This perspective underscores the transformative power inherent in the cultivation of emotional strength.

Example Perspective: Conquering detrimental habits becomes a catalyst for fostering emotional resilience, endowing individuals with the capacity to confront setbacks and challenges with a heightened sense of calmness and adaptability.

5. Sense of Purpose:

- Unearthing or redefining a profound sense of purpose and direction in life emerges as a potent motivator for transformative change.

The recognition that such change aligns personal actions with core values and aspirations amplifies the significance of embarking on this transformative journey.

Personal transformation unfolds as a journey of aligning actions with a deeper sense of purpose, paving the way for a more fulfilling and purpose-driven life. The decisive path to change intricately weaves together the threads of self-awareness, acknowledgment, and motivational insights.

This transformative process empowers individuals to stride confidently into a new chapter of their lives marked by growth, fulfillment, and alignment with their authentic selves.

 In the forthcoming chapters, a detailed exploration of practical strategies will serve as a guiding compass for individuals on this empowering journey   of   change.

Chapter4

Strategies for Overcoming Excessive Masturbation

Embarking on the journey to overcome necessitates a thoughtful fusion of intentional strategies and mindful practices. These intricately designed approaches aspire to cultivate a healthier relationship with one's sexuality and, consequently, play a pivotal role in contributing to overall well-being.

Intentional strategies

1. Cultivating Health-Promoting Habits:

Introducing positive lifestyle changes that bolster both physical and mental well-being is a foundational step. This encompasses the adoption of regular exercise, maintaining a balanced diet, and prioritizing adequate sleep.

Regular engagement in physical activity not only provides a constructive outlet for energy but also plays a crucial role in enhancing mood and overall vitality, diminishing the propensity for excessive masturbation.

2. Avoiding Disturbing Material:

Adopting intentional measures to restrict exposure to explicit or triggering content that could perpetuate the habit of is crucial.

Implementing content filters on devices and practicing mindfulness in media choices contribute to creating an environment that minimizes the likelihood of being influenced by explicit material.

3. Seeking Professional Guidance:

Recognizing the significance of seeking support from healthcare professionals or therapists specializing in sexual health is a pivotal step.

Engaging with a licensed therapist offers personalized guidance, assisting individuals in delving into the root causes of and developing coping mechanisms tailored to their unique circumstances.

4. Practicing Self-Compassion:

Nurturing a compassionate attitude towards oneself, understanding that overcoming habits demands patience and self-kindness, is essential.

Rather than resorting to harsh self-criticism, individuals cultivate the ability to acknowledge progress, celebrate small victories, and approach setbacks with a constructive and compassionate mindset.

Mindful Practices:

1. Awareness of Triggers:

Cultivating a heightened awareness of situations, emotions, or thoughts that trigger the urge for is crucial.

Mindfulness practices empower individuals to identify specific triggers, whether stress, boredom, or loneliness, enabling them to proactively address the underlying issues.

2. Mindful Engagement in Alternative Activities:

Redirecting energy and attention towards alternative, constructive activities that foster personal growth and fulfillment is instrumental.

Cultivating hobbies, pursuing creative endeavors, or engaging in social activities offers positive outlets for energy, diminishing the reliance on excessive masturbation.

3. Establishing Healthy Boundaries:

Embarking on the transformative journey necessitates a profound acknowledgment of the need for change, marking a pivotal step that lays the foundation for embracing a decisive path toward a new and improved reality.

This critical recognition serves as the catalyst for the metamorphosis that follows, propelling individuals towards a more fulfilling and purposeful existence. Let's delve into the key elements of this transformative process, where self-awareness and determination become the guiding forces paving the way for positive change and personal growth.

In the pursuit of a healthy relationship with one's sexuality, it becomes paramount to delve into the nuanced landscape of signs that may indicate excessive masturbation.

This exploration goes beyond the mere physical act, reaching into the realms of emotions and behaviors to offer a comprehensive understanding of an individual's overall well-being.

Recognizing signs on a physical level involves paying attention to the body's responses and cues. These may include changes in energy levels, disruptions in sleep patterns, and potential manifestations of fatigue.

A keen awareness of how the body responds physically to sexual activities provides valuable insights into whether these practices are in harmony with the body's natural rhythms.

Emotional well-being is intricately tied to sexual health. Signs of may manifest as shifts in mood, heightened anxiety, or disproportionate stress responses. Observing these emotional nuances allows individuals to gauge the impact of their sexual practices on their mental and emotional states.

Behaviors often serve as visible markers of underlying issues. Compulsive behaviors, a diminished ability to control the frequency or intensity of masturbation, or neglecting daily responsibilities due to preoccupation with sexual activities are significant behavioral indicators.

Recognizing these changes provides individuals with a mirror to assess whether their sexual practices align with a healthy and balanced lifestyle.

Masturbation triggers the release of neurotransmitters, such as dopamine and serotonin, which contribute to feelings of pleasure and satisfaction. However, frequent and excessive release of these neurotransmitters can lead to their depletion.

This depletion may result in a sense of fatigue as the body struggles to maintain the delicate balance necessary for sustained energy.

The intricate dance of sexual arousal and orgasm orchestrates the release of hormones such as prolactin and oxytocin, contributing to the physiological and emotional aspects of the experience.

Prolactin, known as the "satisfaction hormone," promotes a sense of fulfillment, while oxytocin, often termed the "love hormone," fosters emotional bonding.

However, this delicate hormonal dance can be disrupted through frequent masturbation. Picture these hormones as skilled dancers in perfect harmony during a performance.

With each act of masturbation, there's an increased demand for the release of prolactin and oxytocin.

Now, imagine the dancers being called to perform repeatedly without sufficient intermissions.

The continuous overstimulation of these hormonal responses, especially through frequent masturbation, disrupts the delicate equilibrium that governs their release.

This disruption can lead to an imbalance in hormonal levels, potentially resulting in pervasive fatigue.

In essence, the hormonal system, like a finely tuned orchestra, requires periods of rest and recovery to maintain its delicate balance. Frequent masturbation without adequate intervals for hormonal equilibrium may contribute to a sense of pervasive fatigue, impacting both physical and emotional well-being.

This analogy helps illustrate how the intricate hormonal dance, when disrupted through overstimulation, can play a significant role in influencing the overall energy levels and vitality of an individual.

The physical act of masturbation, coupled with its associated physiological responses, demands a noteworthy amount of energy from the body.

It's akin to engaging in a physical exercise that requires stamina and effort. Just as an athlete needs time to recover after an intense workout, the body also requires recovery time after the energy expenditure involved in masturbation.

Consider the body as an energy bank, and each instance of masturbation as a withdrawal. Without allowing sufficient time for recovery, frequent engagement in this activity can lead to a cumulative depletion of energy resources. This analogy illustrates how, like any physical exertion, masturbation necessitates energy, and an absence of adequate recovery intervals may contribute to an overall sense of energy depletion.

Understanding this dynamic emphasizes the importance of moderation and recognizing the need for the body to restore its energy reserves. It underscores the significance of balancing sexual activities with the body's natural ability to recover, promoting overall well-being and sustained vitality.

Understanding the consequences of excessive masturbation requires examining its acute effects on physical and psychological well-being. In this case, we narrow our focus to one primary outcome: "fatigue and energy expenditure."

This section examines how excessive sex causes physical exhaustion, depletes vital energy, and affects physical and mental processes, affecting overall energy levels. This brief introduction to sex, which overwhelmingly influences both energy levels and well-being, spans many dimensions.

Masturbation acts as a trigger for neurotransmitters, especially dopamine and serotonin, which play an important role in the formation of feelings of pleasure and satisfaction in the brain. These neurotransmitters are important for overall well-being and maintaining a positive state of mind. The most important factor, however, lies in the delicate balance of these neurotransmitters.

Under normal and healthy conditions, the release of dopamine and serotonin leads to feelings of happiness and satisfaction. These neurotransmitters play a role in mood formation, positive reinforcement, and motivation. However, can disrupt this delicate balance. Picture the brain as a finely tuned instrument orchestrating the release of these neurotransmitters in a harmonious symphony. Each act of masturbation demands a surge in dopamine and serotonin, akin to a musical crescendo.

Now, envision this symphony being played incessantly without adequate intermissions. The continuous demand for neurotransmitter release, especially through frequent masturbation, disrupts the intricate balance that governs their function. This disruption can lead to a depletion of these crucial neurotransmitters, contributing to a state of fatigue and mental exhaustion.

Think of it as a pleasure-seeking cycle that, when overstimulated, loses its effectiveness over time. The initial rush of pleasure diminishes, and the individual may find themselves trapped in a cycle of seeking more stimulation to achieve the same level of satisfaction. This cycle can lead to a sense of lethargy and diminished overall energy levels.

Understanding this neurochemical aspect sheds light on how can influence the brain's reward system and impact overall energy and vitality. It emphasizes the importance of moderation, recognizing the need for the brain to recover its neurotransmitter balance for sustained well-being.

In the intricate dance of sexual arousal and orgasm, hormones like prolactin and oxytocin take center stage. Prolactin, often referred to as the "satisfaction hormone," promotes a sense of fulfillment, while oxytocin, known as the "love hormone," fosters emotional bonding.

However, this delicate hormonal dance can be disrupted through frequent masturbation. Picture these hormones as skilled dancers in perfect harmony during a performance. With each act of masturbation, there's an increased demand for the release of prolactin and oxytocin.

Now, imagine the dancers being called to perform repeatedly without sufficient intermissions. The continuous overstimulation of these hormonal responses, especially through frequent masturbation, disrupts the delicate equilibrium that governs their release. This disruption can lead to an imbalance in hormonal levels, potentially resulting in pervasive fatigue.

In essence, the hormonal system, like a finely tuned orchestra, requires periods of rest and recovery to maintain its delicate balance. Frequent masturbation without adequate intervals for hormonal equilibrium may contribute to a sense of pervasive fatigue,

impacting both physical and emotional well-being. This analogy helps illustrate how the intricate hormonal dance, when disrupted through overstimulation, can play a significant role in influencing the overall energy levels and vitality of an individual.

The physical act of masturbation, coupled with its associated physiological responses, demands a noteworthy amount of energy from the body. It's akin to engaging in a physical exercise that requires stamina and effort. Just as an athlete needs time to recover after an intense workout, the body also requires recovery time after the energy expenditure involved in masturbation.

Consider the body as an energy bank, and each instance of masturbation as a withdrawal. Without allowing sufficient time for recovery, frequent engagement in this activity can lead to a cumulative depletion of energy resources. This analogy illustrates how, like any physical exertion, masturbation necessitates energy, and an absence of adequate recovery intervals may contribute to an overall sense of energy depletion.

Understanding this dynamic emphasizes the importance of moderation and recognizing the need for the body to restore its energy reserves. It underscores the significance of balancing sexual activities with the body's natural ability to recover, promoting overall well-being and sustained vitality.

Cultivating Health-Promoting Habits

In the pursuit of a balanced and nourishing lifestyle, individuals are encouraged to adopt health-promoting habits that contribute to their overall well-being. Let's delve into key practices that can support individuals on their journey to overcome excessive masturbation:

1. Establishing Routine:

Establishing a structured daily routine is foundational to reducing impulsive or excessive masturbation. By allocating specific times for work, relaxation, and self-care, individuals can establish a sense of order that minimizes the likelihood of succumbing to compulsive behaviors.

To overcome excessive masturbation, consider implementing a daily routine that includes:

Dedicated Work Hours:

Allocate specific time blocks for work-related activities. Having structured work hours creates a sense of purpose and helps maintain focus on professional responsibilities.

Leisure Time for Hobbies:

- Schedule designated periods for engaging in hobbies and recreational activities. This ensures that individuals have time for enjoyable pursuits beyond work, providing a healthy outlet for relaxation.

Moments of Self-Reflection:

Set aside moments for self-reflection, possibly through mindfulness practices or journaling. This allows individuals to check in with themselves, identify emotional triggers, and proactively address any underlying issues.

This structured approach provides a framework for positive habits and helps mitigate the impulse to engage in excessive masturbation.

By adhering to a well-defined routine, individuals create a balanced and organized environment that promotes overall well-being and reduces the likelihood of succumbing to compulsive behaviors.

2. Regular Physical Exercise:

Engaging in regular physical activity serves as a constructive outlet for energy, reduces stress, and contributes to overall physical well-being. Exercise not only promotes a healthier body but also positively impacts mood and energy levels.

Incorporates regular exercise into her routine, participating in activities such as jogging, yoga, or weightlifting.

This intentional focus on physical well-being not only channels energy positively but also contributes to a more balanced lifestyle, reducing the inclination towards excessive masturbation.

3. Mindful Eating:

Cultivating mindful eating habits involves being conscious of food choices and their impact on overall health, including sexual well-being.

Recognizing the connection between nutrition and sexual health encourages individuals to adopt a balanced and nourishing diet.

To overcome excessive masturbation, becomes mindful of his dietary choices. He includes nutrient-rich foods that support sexual health, such as fruits, vegetables, and whole grains. This intentional approach to nutrition becomes an essential component of his overall well-being.

4. Adequate Sleep:

Prioritizing sufficient and restful sleep is fundamental to enhancing overall energy levels and emotional resilience. Quality sleep not only supports physical recovery but also contributes to mental well-being, reducing stress and fatigue.

Recognizing the importance of sleep in her quest for balanced well-being, establishes a consistent sleep routine. By ensuring she gets adequate rest each night, Emma experiences improved energy levels, heightened emotional resilience, and a decreased inclination towards excessive masturbation.

Avoiding Disturbing Material

1. Content Restriction:

Implementing content restrictions on electronic devices to minimize exposure to explicit or triggering material that may fuel is a prudent strategy. This involves utilizing software or settings that limit access to adult content, creating a digital environment conducive to healthier habits.

By incorporating content filters and restrictions, individuals can reduce the likelihood of encountering stimuli that may trigger excessive masturbation. This proactive approach aligns with the goal of fostering a mindful and intentional relationship with sexual behaviors.

The implementation of content restrictions acts as a practical step in creating a supportive environment that aligns with an individual's desire to overcome excessive masturbation. It adds a layer of control and awareness, contributing to the overall strategy of cultivating a healthier approach to sexual well-being.

2. Mindful Media Consumption:

Being intentional about media choices and opting for content that aligns with health-promoting values is a mindful approach to reduce the likelihood of arousal triggers.

This deliberate decision-making involves selecting media that is in harmony with an individual's well-being goals and minimizing exposure to content that may contribute to excessive masturbation.

By actively choosing content that supports health and avoids explicit or arousing material, individuals create a media environment that aligns with their intentions. This intentional approach contributes to a healthier relationship with sexuality, fostering an environment where media choices are in tune with one's values and goals.

This practice emphasizes the importance of conscious decision-making in shaping the media landscape one engages with, promoting a positive influence on overall well-being. It forms a part of the broader strategy to cultivate a balanced and nourishing lifestyle while overcoming excessive masturbation.

Seeking Professional Guidance

1. Therapeutic Support:

Seeking the guidance of a mental health professional or therapist to explore the root causes of and develop coping strategies is a proactive step toward holistic well-being.

A licensed therapist specializing in sexual health can provide personalized support, offering insights into the psychological aspects contributing to the habit and guiding the individual through effective coping mechanisms.

This intentional seeking of professional assistance emphasizes the value of addressing the underlying factors that may fuel excessive masturbation. Therapeutic sessions create a safe and confidential space for individuals to delve into their thoughts, emotions, and experiences, leading to a better understanding of the habit's origins.

By collaborating with a mental health professional, individuals gain valuable tools to navigate the complexities surrounding and work toward positive change. This approach aligns with the broader strategy of adopting intentional practices to foster a healthier relationship with sexuality and overall well-being.

2. Sexual Health Education:

Engaging in sexual health education or counseling is a proactive measure to gain a deeper understanding of healthy sexual practices and boundaries. This intentional approach involves seeking information and guidance from qualified professionals who specialize in sexual health.

Sexual health education provides individuals with knowledge about the physiological, psychological, and emotional aspects of sexuality. This knowledge empowers individuals to make informed decisions, set boundaries, and foster a positive relationship with their own sexuality.

Counseling, on the other hand, offers a personalized and supportive space for individuals to explore their thoughts, feelings, and behaviors related to sexual health.

A qualified sexual health counselor can assist individuals in identifying and addressing factors contributing to excessive masturbation, providing strategies for moderation and balance.

By actively participating in sexual health education or counseling, individuals embark on a journey of self-discovery and empowerment. This intentional investment in knowledge and support aligns with the overarching goal of cultivating a healthier and more balanced approach to sexuality.

Practicing Self-Compassion

1. Mindfulness and Meditation:

Incorporating mindfulness and meditation practices is a valuable strategy to cultivate self-awareness, reduce stress, and foster a non-judgmental attitude toward oneself.

Mindfulness involves bringing attention to the present moment without judgment, allowing individuals to observe their thoughts and feelings without becoming overwhelmed by them.

By integrating mindfulness and meditation into daily life, individuals create moments of stillness and reflection.

These practices enhance self-awareness, helping individuals recognize triggers and patterns related to excessive masturbation. Mindfulness also promotes a non-judgmental and compassionate attitude, allowing individuals to approach challenges with greater understanding and kindness.

Regular mindfulness and meditation sessions contribute to stress reduction, creating a more balanced mental and emotional state. This increased awareness and emotional resilience support individuals on their journey to overcome by providing tools for self-regulation and coping.

Overall, mindfulness and meditation become integral components of a holistic approach to sexual well-being, promoting self-discovery and fostering a positive relationship with one's sexuality.

2. Positive Affirmations:

Embracing positive affirmations is a powerful practice to counter negative self-perceptions and reinforce a healthy self-image. Affirmations are positive statements that individuals repeat to themselves, aiming to cultivate a positive mindset and reshape negative thought patterns.

In the context of overcoming excessive masturbation, positive affirmations can be tailored to address specific challenges or triggers associated with this behavior.

These affirmations may focus on promoting self-compassion, acknowledging progress, and fostering a positive attitude toward one's sexuality.

For instance, affirmations such as "I am in control of my sexual behaviors," or "I deserve a healthy and balanced relationship with my body" can help shift the internal narrative.

Regularly incorporating positive affirmations into daily routines reinforces a positive self-image and encourages a mindset conducive to change.

By embracing positive affirmations, individuals contribute to building a foundation of self-empowerment and self-love, essential elements for a transformative journey toward a healthier relationship with their sexuality.

3. Developing Coping Mechanisms:

Building healthy coping mechanisms is crucial for managing stress, boredom, or emotional triggers without resorting to excessive masturbation. Coping mechanisms are strategies individuals employ to navigate challenges and emotional distress in a constructive manner.

To cultivate healthier coping mechanisms, individuals can explore alternatives such as mindfulness, exercise, creative activities, or seeking support from friends and family.

These activities serve as positive outlets for stress and help individuals develop resilience in the face of emotional triggers.

For example, engaging in regular physical exercise not only provides a healthy way to release stress but also contributes to improved mood and overall well-being. Similarly, practicing mindfulness techniques, such as meditation or deep breathing exercises, can enhance emotional regulation.

By consciously building and incorporating these healthy coping mechanisms into their daily lives, individuals equip themselves with effective tools to manage challenges, reducing the reliance on as a coping strategy. This proactive approach contributes to a more balanced and resilient lifestyle, fostering overall well-being.

4. Community Support:

Connecting with supportive communities or groups plays a crucial role in overcoming excessive masturbation.

These communities provide individuals with a platform to share their experiences, gain valuable insights, and receive encouragement on their journey toward healthier sexual practices.

For instance, online forums, support groups, or therapy communities focused on sexual health can offer a safe space for individuals to discuss their challenges, share coping strategies, and receive support from others who may be going through similar experiences.

This sense of community fosters a supportive environment that can be instrumental in breaking free from detrimental habits.

By integrating strategies such as connecting with supportive communities into a comprehensive approach, individuals create a powerful and supportive network around them.

This holistic framework, combined with other health-promoting habits and professional guidance, empowers individuals to take proactive steps toward overcoming excessive masturbation. The collective strength of these strategies reinforces a balanced approach to sexuality and contributes to positive and lasting change

Chapter 5.

Navigating Challenges and Setbacks

As individuals embark on the journey to overcome excessive masturbation, they inevitably face challenges and setbacks. This chapter delves into common obstacles that individuals may encounter, offering insights and strategies to navigate these hurdles and maintain progress on the path to positive transformation.

1 Relapse:

Experiencing moments of relapse is a common challenge on this journey. Old habits may resurface, posing a significant obstacle to the progress made. Understanding the nature of relapse and developing strategies to cope with it is essential for sustained growth.

Relapse is a natural part of any transformative journey. It's crucial to approach relapse with understanding rather than judgment. Strategies to cope with relapse may involve self-reflection, seeking support from others, and reassessing the factors that led to the relapse.

2 External Triggers:

Facing external triggers, such as stress or exposure to explicit content, can reignite the impulse for excessive masturbation. Identifying and addressing these triggers is crucial in maintaining control and preventing a return to unhealthy habits.

Recognizing external triggers is the first step in overcoming them. Strategies may involve creating a supportive environment, implementing stress-reduction techniques, and being intentional about media consumption to minimize exposure to triggering content.

3 Negative Emotions:

Coping with negative emotions, such as guilt, shame, or anxiety, is an inherent part of the journey. Acknowledging these emotions and developing healthy coping mechanisms is vital for emotional well-being and continued progress.

Negative emotions are natural responses to challenges. Developing healthy coping mechanisms may include practicing self-compassion, seeking professional support, and engaging in activities that promote emotional well-being.

4 Social Stigma:

Navigating societal or cultural stigma surrounding discussions on masturbation can hinder open communication and support. Overcoming this obstacle involves challenging societal norms and fostering an environment of understanding and empathy.

Addressing social stigma requires courage and a commitment to open dialogue. It involves educating oneself and others about healthy sexuality, promoting empathy, and creating a supportive community that encourages open and judgment-free conversations.

Building Resilience and Perseverance

While setbacks are an inevitable part of the journey, this chapter delves into strategies to navigate challenges with resilience and continue progressing toward positive transformation.

5.2.1 Self-Reflection and Acceptance:

- Engaging in regular self-reflection becomes a cornerstone for understanding the root causes of setbacks. Fostering self-acceptance is recognized as an integral part of the journey, allowing individuals to learn from their experiences without unnecessary self-blame.

Self-reflection involves a deliberate examination of thoughts, emotions, and behaviors, providing valuable insights into the underlying causes of setbacks. Embracing self-acceptance encourages a compassionate view of oneself, acknowledging that setbacks are part of the growth process.

5.2.2 Learning from Setbacks:

Setbacks are reframed as opportunities for learning and growth rather than failures. Extracting valuable insights from each setback becomes a crucial skill, empowering individuals with the knowledge needed for future resilience.

Each setback offers a unique opportunity to gather insights into personal triggers, vulnerabilities, and areas that require additional focus. By reframing setbacks as valuable learning experiences, individuals gain a deeper understanding of themselves and their journey.

5.2.3 Adapting Strategies:

Flexibility in adapting and refining strategies based on personal experiences ensures a dynamic and evolving approach to overcoming challenges. This adaptive mindset empowers individuals to tailor their strategies for maximum effectiveness.

Adapting strategies involves a continuous assessment of what works and what needs adjustment. It requires a willingness to experiment with different approaches, embracing the idea that personal growth is a fluid and evolving process. This adaptability ensures a personalized and effective response to challenges.

In navigating setbacks, building resilience, and persevering through challenges become integral aspects of the transformative journey. These strategies provide a robust framework for individuals not only to overcome obstacles but also to use setbacks as stepping stones toward lasting positive change.

encouragement during challenging times.

5.2.4. Professional Guidance:

Seeking the guidance of mental health professionals or therapists is emphasized to navigate emotional challenges and receive expert advice tailored to individual needs. The expertise of these professionals becomes a valuable resource in the transformative process.

5.2 5. Mindfulness Practices:

Incorporating mindfulness practices becomes a powerful tool for staying present in the moment, managing stress, and avoiding overwhelm during setbacks. Mindfulness fosters a heightened awareness that can positively impact decision-making and behavior.

5.2.6 Setting Realistic Expectations:

Establishing realistic expectations is vital, recognizing that the journey toward overcoming is a gradual and iterative process. Setting achievable goals ensures that individuals remain motivated and committed to sustainable change.

5.2.7 Celebrating Progress:

Celebrating small victories and recognizing the progress made becomes a cornerstone for fostering a positive mindset and sustaining motivation throughout the journey.

Acknowledging achievements, no matter how small, contributes to a sense of accomplishment.

Chapter 6.

The Positive Outcomes of Abandoning Excessive Masturbation

As individuals commit to abandoning excessive masturbation, they unlock a spectrum of positive outcomes that extend across various dimensions of their lives.

Embracing a healthier relationship with sexuality leads to transformative changes, fostering improved physical health, enhanced mental well-being, and rejuvenated relationships.

6.1 Improved Physical Health

There are many health benefits that comes with stopping excessive masturbation.

6.1.1 Increased Energy Levels:

Abandoning contributes to reduced energy depletion, resulting in increased vitality and overall physical stamina.

Excessive masturbation, with its associated physical and physiological demands, often leads to energy depletion. As individuals break free from this pattern, they experience a noticeable increase in energy levels.

This surge in vitality enables them to engage more actively in daily activities, fostering an overall sense of well-being. Regular engagement in healthy habits, such as exercise and balanced nutrition, further complements this newfound energy, creating a positive cycle of physical wellness.

6.1.2 Enhanced Physical Stamina:

The cessation of allows the body to recover and rejuvenate, contributing to improved physical stamina and endurance.

Excessive sexual activity can strain the body, leading to physical fatigue and reduced stamina. Abandoning this habit provides the body with the necessary time and resources to recover.

Individuals may notice enhanced physical stamina and endurance, making activities that once felt draining more manageable. This improvement in physical resilience is a direct result of the body's ability to restore itself when freed from the persistent demands of excessive masturbation.

6.1.3 Better Sleep Quality:

Breaking free from the cycle of often leads to improved sleep quality, fostering overall physical health.

Excessive sexual activity, especially close to bedtime, can disrupt sleep patterns.

Abandoning this habit contributes to better sleep quality, allowing the body to enter restorative sleep phases. Improved sleep, in turn, enhances physical health by supporting processes such as muscle repair, immune function, and hormonal balance.

As individuals experience more restful sleep, they further contribute to their overall physical well-being.

6.1.4 Enhanced Immune Function:

The reduction of physical and psychological stress associated with positively impacts immune function, leading to a stronger and more resilient immune system.

Frequent engagement in can contribute to elevated stress levels, impacting immune function. By abandoning this habit, individuals experience a reduction in both physical and psychological stress.

This in turn, supports a more robust immune system. A strengthened immune function enhances the body's ability to defend against illnesses, contributing significantly to improved overall physical health.

6.2. Enhanced Mental Well-being

6.2.1 Reduced Stress and Anxiety:

Abandoning detrimental habits alleviates stress and anxiety associated with excessive masturbation, fostering a more relaxed and composed mental state.

can contribute to heightened stress and anxiety levels, impacting an individual's overall mental well-being. By breaking free from this compulsive cycle, individuals experience a notable reduction in stress and anxiety.

The absence of guilt or shame associated with excessive sexual activity allows for a more serene mental state. This newfound calmness forms a solid foundation for improved mental health, positively influencing various aspects of daily life.

6.2.2 Improved Cognitive Function:

A healthier relationship with sexuality contributes to improved cognitive function, including better focus, concentration, and mental clarity.

Excessive sexual activity, especially when compulsive, can interfere with cognitive function. Abandoning this habit allows individuals to reclaim mental clarity, enhancing their ability to focus and concentrate. Improved cognitive function positively influences productivity, problem-solving skills, and overall mental acuity. As individuals embrace a healthier relationship with their sexuality, they often find that their mental faculties become more resilient and responsive.

6.2.3 Elevated Mood:

Breaking free from the compulsive cycle of often leads to a significant improvement in mood, fostering a more positive and optimistic outlook on life.

The habitual nature of can contribute to mood swings and fluctuations. Abandoning this cycle allows individuals to experience a sustained improvement in mood.

The release from guilt, anxiety, and the addictive nature of the behavior contributes to an overall positive outlook on life. Elevated mood becomes a natural outcome of the mental and emotional liberation that accompanies the decision to abandon excessive masturbation.

6.3 Emotional Liberation:

Liberation from the compulsive habits associated with allows individuals to break free from the emotional burdens that may accompany it. This newfound freedom contributes to an elevated mood as the individual experiences a sense of release from negative emotions such as guilt, shame, or anxiety.

6.3.1 Hormonal Balance:

- The cessation of contributes to the restoration of hormonal balance. Hormones play a crucial role in regulating mood, and when this balance is restored, individuals often report feeling more stable emotionally. This positive hormonal shift can contribute to an overall improvement in mood.

Hormones, including serotonin, dopamine, and oxytocin, influence mood and emotional well-being. can disrupt this delicate hormonal balance, leading to mood swings and emotional instability.

Abandoning allows the body to regain hormonal equilibrium, fostering emotional stability. As hormones stabilize, individuals may find themselves better equipped to manage stressors and experience a more consistent and positive mood.

6.3.2 Increased Dopamine Sensitivity:

It can lead to a desensitization of dopamine receptors, the neurotransmitter associated with pleasure and reward. Breaking free from this compulsive cycle allows for the restoration of dopamine sensitivity, leading to an increased capacity for experiencing joy and positive emotions.

Dopamine is a key neurotransmitter that regulates pleasure and reward. Overstimulation from can lead to a decrease in dopamine sensitivity, making it challenging to experience pleasure from everyday activities.

Abandoning allows the brain's reward system to reset, restoring sensitivity to dopamine. This heightened sensitivity contributes to an increased capacity for joy, satisfaction, and positive emotions in response to various stimuli.

6.3.3 Reduced Stress and Anxiety:

It is often linked to increased stress and anxiety levels. By breaking free from this cycle, individuals can experience a reduction in stress and anxiety, creating a conducive environment for an elevated mood.

Chronic engagement in can lead to heightened stress and anxiety due to factors such as guilt, shame, or the impact of hormonal fluctuations. Abandoning this compulsive behavior provides relief from these stressors, allowing individuals to experience a noticeable reduction in overall stress and anxiety levels.

As stress diminishes, a more relaxed and serene state of mind emerges, contributing to an elevated and positive mood.

6.4 Positive Self-Perception.

The act of overcoming a challenging habit fosters a positive self-perception. Individuals may experience a boost in self-esteem and self-confidence, contributing to a more positive overall outlook on life.

Improved Interpersonal Relationships.

As mood improves, individuals may find it easier to engage positively in interpersonal relationships.

Healthy connections and social interactions further contribute to a positive and optimistic perspective.

In essence, the elevation in mood following the decision to break free from is a multifaceted transformation that involves emotional liberation, hormonal balance, increased dopamine sensitivity, stress reduction, positive self-perception, and improved interpersonal relationships.

It marks a pivotal aspect of the holistic well-being that individuals can achieve on their journey towards a healthier and more balanced life.4. Greater Emotional Resilience.

Embracing a balanced sexual lifestyle enhances emotional resilience, empowering individuals to navigate life's challenges with greater ease.

Rejuvenated Relationships

1. Enhanced Intimacy:

Abandoning paves the way for a more intimate and fulfilling connection with a partner, fostering a deeper emotional bond.

2. Improved Communication:

A healthier approach to sexual habits often correlates with improved communication within relationships, creating a more open and understanding dynamic.

3. Increased Relationship Satisfaction:

Breaking free from the negative impacts of contributes to an overall increase in relationship satisfaction and mutual well-being.

4. Greater Emotional Availability:

Ceasing detrimental habits allows individuals to be more emotionally available, promoting a supportive and nurturing environment within relationships.

Embracing the positive outcomes of abandoning transcends the individual, creating a ripple effect that influences physical health, mental well-being, and the quality of relationships. As individuals navigate this transformative journey, they discover a path toward holistic well-being and the fulfillment of their personal and relational potentials.

Chapter 7.

Embracing a Balanced Lifestyle

As individuals transition towards abandoning excessive masturbation, the journey involves not just cessation but the active cultivation of a balanced lifestyle. This holistic approach encompasses the cultivation of healthy habits and the discovery of fulfillment beyond the realm of masturbation.

7.1 Cultivating Healthy Habits

7.1.1 Mindful Self-Care:

- Fostering connections with supportive communities or individuals who share similar goals and values.

Building connections with others on a similar journey provides a sense of community and mutual support. Sharing experiences, insights, and encouragement with like-minded individuals fosters a supportive environment.

This network can serve as a valuable resource during challenging times, offering understanding, empathy, and motivation. By actively participating in a supportive community, individuals enhance their resilience and create lasting connections that contribute to overall well-being.

7.1.2 Establishing Boundaries:

Cultivating mindfulness practices to stay present in the moment and develop a heightened awareness of thoughts and emotions.

Mindfulness plays a crucial role in maintaining a balanced lifestyle. By cultivating awareness of thoughts and emotions, individuals can identify potential triggers and address them proactively. Mindfulness practices, such as meditation and deep breathing, contribute to emotional regulation and stress reduction.

Staying present in the moment enhances overall well-being and helps individuals navigate challenges with greater resilience. The incorporation of mindfulness into daily life fosters a holistic approach to health and supports the ongoing journey toward positive transformation.

7.1.3 Mindfulness and Meditation:

Embarking on a transformative journey to overcome involves not only understanding the challenges and setbacks but also actively cultivating strategies for lasting change. This chapter explores practical approaches and habits that individuals can adopt to support their ongoing journey toward a healthier relationship with sexuality and overall well-being.

7.1.4 Regular Physical Exercise:

Nurturing supportive relationships and open communication with trusted individuals, such as friends, family, or a supportive community.

Building a support network is essential for the journey toward overcoming excessive masturbation.

Trusted individuals can provide understanding, encouragement, and accountability. Open communication fosters an environment where challenges and successes can be shared without judgment, creating a supportive space for growth.

By cultivating meaningful connections, individuals strengthen their resolve and create a network that reinforces positive change.

7.2 Exploring Hobbies and Interests:

7.2.1 Actively Exploring and Pursuing:

Embracing ongoing self-education on sexual health, healthy relationships, and the broader aspects of well-being.

Continuous learning about sexual health and healthy relationships is a vital aspect of the transformative journey. By staying informed, individuals empower themselves with knowledge that supports positive decision-making and reinforces a balanced approach to sexuality.

Ongoing self-education fosters a deeper understanding of the intricate connections between physical, mental, and emotional well-being, contributing to sustained personal growth and overall transformation.

7.3 Cultivating Social Connections:

7.3.1 Nurturing Social Connections:

Nurturing social connections and building meaningful relationships with friends, family, and the community to create a supportive network.

Social connections play a crucial role in maintaining a balanced lifestyle. Building meaningful relationships provides emotional support, reduces feelings of isolation, and creates a network of individuals who can offer encouragement and understanding.

Nurturing social connections contributes to a sense of belonging and reinforces the commitment to positive habits.

7.4 Personal Growth and Learning:

7.4.1 Investing Time in Personal Growth:

Investing time in personal growth and continuous learning, whether through formal education, reading, or skill development, to enhance one's sense of purpose.

Continuous learning and personal growth contribute to an individual's sense of purpose and fulfillment. Whether pursuing formal education, reading books, or developing new skills, these endeavors foster intellectual stimulation and personal development.

Investing time in personal growth aligns with a commitment to positive change and creates a foundation for a more meaningful life.

7.5 Setting and Achieving Goals:

7.5.1 Establishing Realistic and Achievable Goals:

Establishing realistic and achievable goals, both short-term and long-term, to provide direction and motivation in life beyond the immediate challenges.

Goal-setting provides individuals with a sense of direction and purpose. Establishing both short-term and long-term goals creates a roadmap for personal development.

Achieving these goals boosts confidence, reinforces positive habits, and serves as a constant source of motivation throughout the journey.

7.6 Spiritual Exploration:

7.6.1 Exploring Spiritual Practices:

Exploring spiritual practices or engaging in contemplative activities that resonate with personal beliefs, contributing to a deeper sense of purpose and connection.

Spiritual exploration goes beyond religious affiliations. It involves engaging in activities that foster a sense of connection with something greater than oneself.

Whether through meditation, mindfulness, or specific religious practices, spiritual exploration provides a deeper understanding of purpose and can be a source of solace and guidance.

7.7 Embracing Emotional Well-being:

7.7.1 Prioritizing Emotional Well-being:

Prioritizing emotional well-being by seeking therapy, participating in support groups, or practicing self-reflection to navigate and understand emotions more effectively.

Prioritizing emotional well-being involves acknowledging and understanding emotions. Seeking therapy or participating in support groups provides a structured and supportive environment for emotional exploration.

Practicing self-reflection enhances emotional intelligence, empowering individuals to navigate challenges with resilience and self-awareness.

7.8 Cultivating Healthy Relationships:

7.8.1 Focusing on Building and Maintaining:

Focusing on building and maintaining healthy relationships, both romantic and platonic, to foster a supportive and enriching social environment.

Healthy relationships are vital for overall well-being. Focusing on building and maintaining positive connections with others creates a supportive social environment.

Nurturing healthy relationships involves effective communication, empathy, and mutual support, reinforcing a positive and balanced lifestyle.

Embracing a balanced lifestyle extends beyond the absence of detrimental habits. Actively exploring hobbies, nurturing social connections, investing in personal growth, setting achievable goals, exploring spirituality, prioritizing emotional well-being, and cultivating healthy relationships collectively contribute to a holistic and fulfilling life.

These aspects form a comprehensive approach to maintaining positive changes and achieving lasting well-being.

Chapter 8:

Conclusion

In concluding the transformative journey of abandoning excessive masturbation, it is imperative to reflect on the long-term benefits of breaking free and to celebrate the profound personal growth and transformation achieved.

The Long-Term Benefits of Breaking Free

8.1 Holistic Well-being:

Achieving a state of holistic well-being that encompasses physical health, mental clarity, emotional resilience, and enhanced relational dynamics.

Holistic well-being signifies a comprehensive state of health that goes beyond the absence of detrimental habits. It involves nurturing physical health, fostering mental clarity, building emotional resilience, and cultivating positive relationships. This multifaceted approach creates a foundation for sustained well-being.

8.2 Renewed Energy and Vitality:

Experiencing a renewed sense of energy and vitality as the body and mind recover from the impacts of excessive masturbation.

Breaking free from the cycle of allows the body and mind to undergo a process of rejuvenation. As energy resources are replenished, individuals experience increased vitality and a restored sense of vigor, contributing to a more energetic and vibrant lifestyle.

8.3 Improved Relationships:

Fostering improved relationships, marked by increased intimacy, communication, and mutual satisfaction.

Overcoming positively impacts relational dynamics.

Increased intimacy, open communication, and mutual satisfaction become integral components of improved relationships.

Breaking free from detrimental habits allows individuals to invest more time and energy in building meaningful connections.

8.4 Emotional Liberation:

Attaining emotional liberation from the negative cycles associated with excessive masturbation, leading to a more positive and balanced emotional state.

Emotional liberation involves breaking free from negative cycles and achieving a balanced emotional state. Individuals experience a sense of freedom from guilt, shame, and anxiety, fostering emotional well-being and contributing to a more positive outlook on life.

8.5 Personal Fulfillment:

Discovering personal fulfillment beyond the confines of detrimental habits, finding joy and purpose in a more balanced and meaningful life.

Personal fulfillment arises from aligning actions with core values and aspirations. Breaking free from allows individuals to discover joy, purpose, and fulfillment in activities that contribute to a more balanced and meaningful life.

www.ingramcontent.com/pod-product-compliance
Lightning Source LLC
Chambersburg PA
CBHW050817260726
48660CB00004B/1489